FIT FOR PRAYER

LEARN HOW TO FIT PRAYER AND PHYSICAL ACTIVITY INTO YOUR DAILY ROUTINE

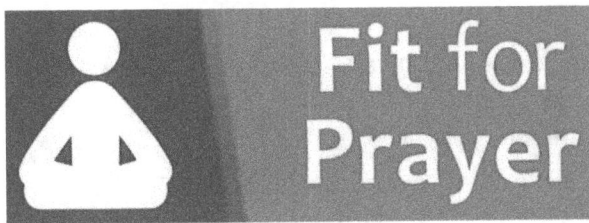

KIMBERLEY PAYNE

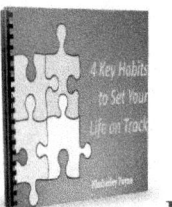

Free Report Reveals…
The 4 Key Habits to Set your Life on Track

7 health & fitness experts share their top spiritual & physical health tips.

Learn quick tips to improve your daily habits in Bible study, eating healthy, exercise and prayer.

Visit www.kimberleypayne.com/free-report
to download your free report today!

Table of Contents

Introduction

Congratulations! You have made an important step towards a healthier you.

Fit for Prayer unites physical health and spiritual health to help you lose weight and develop a deeper relationship with God. You will gain insight into how to incorporate prayer and fitness into your daily routine.

God created you as a whole person, therefore, take care of your whole self, not just the individual parts. A direct relationship exists between physical, emotional and spiritual health. A healthy body gives you the energy and enthusiasm to carry out the purposes that God has for your life. Practicing healthy living glorifies God.

Exercise your body + Exercise your spirit

Cardiovascular exercise & Strength training + Prayer

Think of exercise as either cardiovascular activity or strength training. Cardiovascular activity helps you to increase energy and keep moving. It's good for your heart, lungs and circulatory system. Strength training (also known as weightlifting) helps you keep your bones and muscles strong, reduces bone loss, and improves balance and posture.

Prayer helps you to enter into a spiritual communion with God.

What cardiovascular exercise and strength training do for building a strong body, prayer does to build spiritual strength. Your body requires exercise and food, and it needs these things regularly. You cannot just take care of it at the beginning of the week and forget about it. Your spiritual life is similar to your physical body in that way. You cannot pray just once and have a healthy, growing spiritual life.

Just as exercise strengthens your body, prayer strengthens your spirit. Similarities between exercise and prayer include:

- To be physically and spiritually healthy requires discipline. You need to practice both daily and use this strength or you will lose it.

- The effects can be both immediate and/or long term. You may see the results right away or the effects can be cumulative.

- Both exercise and prayer improve balance in your life, improve your quality of life and boost your mood.

- With a pure motive, both delight God.

Chapter 1: Exercise your Body

What it is
Don't you know that you yourselves are God's temple and that God's Spirit lives in you? (1 Corinthians 3:16)

Exercise rejuvenates your body. Cardiovascular exercise equips you to sustain an activity for a long period of time. It causes you to breathe more deeply and work your heart harder. When you are strength training you use resistance to strengthen your muscles.

What it's not

Cardiovascular exercise is not only going to the gym and participating in an aerobics class. It does not make any difference whether you go to a gym or what equipment you use. Try to figure out where activity fits into your life. Any physical activity is better than no exercise. You need to do only about 30 minutes of moderate exercise daily and that half-hour can accumulate in shorter pieces.

Strength training is not only for men or for younger people. Women of any age can also benefit, particularly those most likely to suffer from osteoporosis.

Benefits of exercise

- Elevates mood
- Improves balance and mobility
- Maintains a healthy weight
- Increases energy level

- Builds strength and tones muscles
- A pure motive delights God

Discover the many benefits to exercise, including feelings of accomplishment and well-being, increased energy, reduced stress and improved sleep patterns. Research indicates that activity reduces the risk of heart disease, falls and injuries, obesity, high blood pressure, adult onset diabetes, osteoporosis, stroke, depression, colon cancer and premature death. The U.S. Surgeon General has determined that lack of physical activity is as detrimental to your health as smoking a pack of cigarettes a day.

Regular cardiovascular exercise (aerobic exercise) helps you burn calories faster, even when you are sitting still. It does this by raising your metabolism (the rate you burn calories) up to 15 hours after exercising.

Strength training (weight lifting) helps you to better deal with every day tasks, improves posture, increases firmness of muscles, and helps prevent osteoporosis. It also helps you build muscle so that even if you do not lose pounds, you may lose inches.

You need to include both cardiovascular exercise as well as strength training into your exercise program.

Chapter 2: Exercise Strategies that Work

Take it slow and steady
Remember that fitness is not a "quick fix". With a lifestyle change you may experience setbacks and plateaus. Think of this program as a start to a whole new lifestyle.

Schedule exercise in
Take an honest look at how you spend your days. Schedule exercise in your daily planner just as you would a business meeting or a doctor's appointment.

Track your progress
Keep a chart of your progress and take notice of small improvements.

Follow the 10-minute rule
Decide to do only 10 minutes of exercise and then you can stop if you want. Generally, once you start exercising you will not want to stop.

Team up with a friend
A partner can make workouts more fun and push you to try harder. You will be more likely to stick to your plan if you have a partner. Join a walking club, a sports team or an aerobics class.

Do something else at the same time
You can read or listen to books on tape while riding a stationary bike. You can also watch TV, listen to music, talk to God or think about the Scripture reading. If

outdoors, carry a trash bag with you and collect garbage along the road or trail.

Create space
Create an area to call your own and make exercise so accessible that you have no excuse. Buy some low-priced equipment: an exercise bike, a resistance band, a set of dumbells, a stretching mat, a jump rope and an exercise video.

Look the part
Put on workout clothes – do not just change into running shoes. If you look the part, you will feel the part. Keep workout clothes in the car or beside the front door.

Time it right
Remember, if you do not have the time for a full workout each day, break down your workouts into three or four smaller chunks of 10 minutes each. You can do different things in each of these times.

Vary your routine
You may be less likely to get bored or injured if you change your routine. Walk one day and bicycle the next.

Have fun
Take the "work" out of workouts. Try something new and experiment until you find one that you like doing. The best fitness plan is one that you can easily include in your busy schedule.

Celebrate goals reached
Every time you reach a goal, celebrate. Reward ideas may
include making a long-distance phone call, treating yourself
to a long bubble bath, getting a pedicure, facial or massage,
buying an extravagant bouquet, or subscribing to an
exercise magazine.

Make fitness a family activity
Plan a weekend hike, sign up for line-dancing together,
coach your child's sports team, go ice-skating at the local
community centre, plan a canoeing vacation, take an after-
dinner walk, sign up for a mother-and-child exercise class,
or go sledding together.

Learn to include simple activities into your daily routine.
Park your vehicle over a block away from work. Once at
work, favor the stairs over the elevator. Pull out your
bicycle and ride to pick up your mail. Roller-blade around
the neighborhood with the family dog. Hike through the
fields and pick wild flowers to make floral arrangements
for gifts. Join the children after school for a session of jump
rope skipping or smash a birdie over the backyard
badminton net.

If your schedule is full of everyone else's extra-curricular
activities, incorporate personal fitness during these times.
For example, kick the ball around the field at your child's
soccer tournament. Or toss a ball on the sidelines at your
spouse's baseball game. You may want to help out a
worthy cause by joining a walk-a-thon. A mother-daughter
walk is an example of one way to combine fitness with
family bonding.

Walking is one of the most flexible and relaxing activities. You do not need any special equipment or skills – just a good pair of shoes and sensible clothing. You can do it anywhere and anytime with a friend or by yourself. Walking offers less risk of injury, with many of the benefits of more strenuous activities.

Chapter 3: Exercise Goal Planning

How do you get started?

Talk with your doctor
You should get medical clearance from your physician before making any significant changes in your physical activity level.

Set a goal
What are the benefits of setting goals? Goals give you the direction, energy and purpose you need to get going. Goals decrease stress and give you a sense of control and accomplishment.

There are two questions to answer when setting and achieving goals:
1. What is your goal?
2. How do you reach your goal?

1.What is your goal?

Finding your fit level establishes your starting point. It shows you where you need improvement and it can help you to chart your progress.

Goals need to be specific. A vague goal is unlikely to be accomplished. First, a complex or long-term goal needs to be broken down into smaller or shorter-term goals to ensure success. Then, the way to know whether you have accomplished your goal is if you have some way to measure it. Ideally you can use numbers to track your progress and achievement. (See examples below) Thirdly, to ensure success, make your goal attainable and achievable. Lastly, without a realistic deadline it is too easy to procrastinate. A time limit will help you stay focused on your goal.

Examples:

To say, "I want to lose weight" isn't specific enough. To say, "I want to lose 100 pounds in three weeks" lacks realism. Instead a more specific and realistic goal starts, "I will lose 10 pounds in two months."

"I will lose two inches from my thighs in three months."

"I will compete in a marathon this autumn."

"I will be strong enough to pick up my two-year old before he turns three."

"I will walk up the 40 stairs at work without feeling winded by December."

"I will cycle three miles to the grocery store by the end of the month."

You get the idea.

2. How do you reach your goal?

There are four major variables to consider when setting up a fitness program. A well-designed program follows the FITT formula: Frequency, Intensity, Time, and Type.

A. Frequency

Think of frequency as the number of cardiovascular exercise training sessions per week. You can exercise every day of the week with one day set aside for rest. By taking one day off each week, you will come back to your activity feeling stronger and more energetic.

Aim to strength train two to three times per week on alternate days. Set aside at least 48 hours to allow your muscles to fully recover.

B. Intensity

In cardiovascular exercise, intensity asks, "How hard are you working?" Choose activities that raise your heart and breathing rates. Use the Talk Test as a simple way to monitor your exercise intensity. You should always be able to hold a conversation while exercising. Adjust exercise intensity to make two to three-word phrases possible.

Pay attention to signs of overexertion, such as pounding in your chest, dizziness or faintness, or profuse sweating. Cool down for five to ten minutes before ending your workout. If any symptoms persist, see your doctor.

In strength training, intensity refers to the speed or workload (resistance) of exercise. Lift weights heavy enough to complete the last few repetitions of each set, but not so tough that you compromise your form.

C. Time

Time in the FITT formula relates to the duration of the workout. For health benefits, try to perform 30 minutes of cardiovascular exercise every day. You can break down your activity into smaller chunks of time. Think about times that you can do physical activity for ten minutes and build up to 30 minutes.

With strength training, the length of the workout depends on the result desired. You do not need to spend hours in a gym. You can have an effective workout in just 30 minutes. However, lift the weights slowly.

D. Type

The best type of cardiovascular exercise is any exercise that you will keep doing throughout your life. You must enjoy the activity you choose. Just be sure that when creating your program, you first consult your physician.

Think about activities that you participated in before, are currently involved in, or would like to try. Activities may include:

- Aerobics, alpine skiing, aquatics

- Ballet, basketball, baseball, badminton, bicycling

- Canoeing, cross-country skiing, curling

- Dance, gardening, golf, hiking

- Ice hockey, ice-skating, in-line skating

- Jogging, kayaking

- Racquetball, rock climbing, running, rowing

- Soccer, squash, step aerobics, swimming

- Tennis, treadmill, volleyball, walking

Other: _____

With strength training, the type of exercise determines the outcome of your training program. It is important to have an overall development of the body and perform exercises in the order of larger muscle groups to smaller ones. Start with your legs, back and chest. Then work smaller muscles – shoulders, arms, and abdomen. Do the toughest exercises when you are least tired.

There are plenty of workout programs to follow. When designing goals think about the steps necessary to achieve these goals. As well, pick a reasonable time frame for achieving these goals and decide how you will measure progress.

Examples:

Goal: Lose 10 pounds and 2 inches off my waist
Time: Ten weeks (1 pound per week)

Steps:
1. Take measurements and weigh in
2. Interval training: Swim daily and bike 6x per week for 45 minutes
3. Nutrition analysis: track my eating for one week and reduce calorie intake
4. Strength train a minimum of 2x per week

Progress: Changes in the scale and improvement in measurements

Goal: Improve cardiovascular fitness and reduce risk of heart disease
Time: Seven weeks

Steps:
1. Stationary biking 4x per week or walk 30 minutes at moderate intensity
2. Outdoor cycling to work (10 km) daily
3. Buy new bike

Progress: Bike 100 miles

Now it's your turn:

Goal:
Time:

Steps: 1.

        2.

        3.

Progress:

Goal:
Time:

Steps: 1.

        2.

        3.

Progress:

Think about...

1. What is the lowest weight you have maintained as an adult for one year? What is the largest clothes size you feel comfortable in?

2. Do you have the support of your family?

3. What equipment do you presently have access to? Are you willing to spend money on equipment and supplies?

4. Where can you participate in the activities you enjoy?

5. How do you see your life being different when you meet your goals?

Chapter 4: Exercise your Spirit

What it is

Do not be anxious about anything, but in everything, by prayer and petition, with thanksgiving, present your requests to God. And the peace of God, which transcends all understanding, will guard your hearts and your minds in Christ Jesus. (Philippians 4:6)

Prayer builds your spiritual strength. It can include praise, confession, thanksgiving or appeal. Prayer puts you in contact with God, Who has more power than you could ever imagine. When you pray, He hears you and fills you with the power to do things you never thought you could do.

What it's not

Prayer is not just for highly-spiritual people. God delights to have you come to Him with your requests. You do not have to be "good enough" to pray.

Like exercise, prayer is not a one-time thing. You can pray every day, anywhere and anytime. It is important to spend time in private prayer each day–just you and God.

Prayer is not talking to others, reading or studying. It is not "doing" something. You need to let everything inside you get still. You may feel compelled to cram every moment with activities and external stimuli. Still your mind and listen for God's voice to emerge. (Psalm 46:10)

Prayer is not just about you talking to God, but God talking to you. With prayer you can have a private audience with the Lord. An intimate dialogue goes on inside where there may not be an audible voice, but Spirit to spirit.

Benefits of prayer

- Allows intimate dialogue with God
- Encourages you to face a new day
- Provides information and strategies
- Accomplishes the impossible
- Develops deeper relationship
- A pure motive delights God

Prayer, when combined with quiet time, can decrease respiratory rate, heart rate, elevated blood pressure and muscle tension. During prayer, the body escapes from the stresses of every day life and enters into a relaxed state.

Chapter 5: Prayer Strategies That Work

Follow the P.A.T.H. (praise, admit, thank, help) to prayer:

Praise
Worship the Lord with gladness; come before Him with joyful songs. (Psalm 100:2)

Recognize God and His greatness. Give Him praise and honor. This takes the focus off why you are praying and puts it on the One who can answer. Focus on God first, and the problem diminishes. Your praises should outweigh your petitions. If you do not know what to praise God for, explore His attributes and character from the Bible. Based on your personal history, or past negative experiences, you may have to change some of your thoughts about God.

Admit
Have mercy on me, O God, according to Your unfailing love…blot out my transgressions. Wash away all my iniquity and cleanse me from my sin. (Psalm 51:1-2)

Admit you did wrong. Be repentant and confess your sin. Do not try to hide your sins or failures, but do not dwell on them either. Be honest, God knows. God will give you a way of escape from every temptation. Ask for God's forgiveness, strength and help. His strength is made perfect in your weakness. Admit that His forgiveness of your sin is effective.

Thank
Give thanks to the Lord, for He is good. (Psalm 136:1)

Verbalize what you are grateful for. Make it a personal expression of your heart and an individual connection. Hold nothing back. Use passion. You are invited to gain an understanding that much of what is good in life is a result of God's creative goodness. Sometimes people tend to blame God for the bad in life, and seldom consider that He authors all good.

Help
So I say to you: Ask and it will be given to you; seek and you will find; knock and the door will be opened to you. For everyone who asks receives; he who seeks finds; and to him who knocks, the door will be opened. (Luke 11:9-10)

Bring all your requests – spiritual, emotional, physical and material – to God in prayer. Rely on the fact that God has a faithful and generous nature, always seeking your best. God wants to give you the desires of your heart according to His plan. You need not take things on in your own strength. You need only ask. Nothing is too big or too small to bring to God. He wants you to glorify His name. You can ask for good weather on the weekend, to find your keys in a marsh, or to help you to lose ten pounds, it does not matter. God knows that all your needs are important to you.

Chapter 6: Prayer Goal Planning

God does hear your prayers and He does answer them (although sometimes His answer is No). God is all-powerful. God not only answers your prayers, He provides you with information about your strengths and weaknesses, techniques for solving problems and encouragement to face the day.

In strength training, you start by lifting small weights, and as you grow stronger, you can lift heavier weights. It is the same with prayer. You start by praying a short amount of time, and then as your desire grows, you can plan to spend time in prayer every day.

It is important not only to find time for prayer but also to make time. You need to seek God daily. Every day you can ask for God's help. God wants to help you.

Now it's your turn to make a list of goals that will help you improve your prayer life:

1.

2.

3.

Think about…

1. How much time each day are you currently praying?

2. With whom do you/would you usually pray?

3. How much time are you able to commit to prayer?

4. When would be an inspiring time to pray?

5. Where would be a quiet place to pray?

Chapter 7: Test Your Knowledge

Test your knowledge with these true or false questions.

Frequency (how often)

T or F I have no time to exercise.

T or F I must pray only in the mornings.

T or F I should work out hard during a cold or flu.

T or F I have no time for prayer.

T or F There is no such thing as exercising too much.

Intensity (how hard)

T or F Low-intensity exercise will not promote weight loss like high-intensity.

T or F Prayer is only for highly spiritual people.

T or F Muscle soreness is a sign of a good workout, "No pain, no gain."

T or F I must be busy with talking, reading or studying during prayer time.

T or F I should continue working out even if I hurt myself.

Time (how long)

T or F I need to spend hours in the gym to see results from an exercise program.

T or F I must pray for at least one hour at a time.

T or F I have to work out for at least 30 minutes at a time for health benefits.

Type (how to exercise)

T or F If women lift weights they will bulk up.

T or F There is only one way to say my prayers.

T or F I need specialized equipment to weight train.

T or F I must say the same prayer each day.

T or F I shouldn't start strength training until I am within 25 pounds of my ideal weight.

Answers to True or False questions:

Frequency (how often)

F: I have no time to exercise.
Truth: Exercise means active living. You can walk your dog or take the stairs instead of an elevator. For a more formal program, schedule time for yourself to exercise with the same amount of respect and consideration that you would schedule an appointment with your doctor.

F: I must pray only in the mornings.
Truth: Like exercise, prayer is not a one-time thing. You can pray every day, anywhere and anytime.

F: I should work out hard during a cold or flu.
Truth: Your body tries to fight an illness and if you overtax it with strenuous exercise you could run the risk of getting sicker. Once you're better, use shorter, less intense sessions to build slowly back up to your former level.

F: I have no time for prayer.
Truth: It is important not only to find time for prayer, but to make time. You need to seek God daily. God does not want you to help yourself; He wants to help you.

F: There is no such thing as exercising too much.
Truth: If you exercise too much your body will hold onto its main resource of fuel, which is fat. Also, exercising too much compromises your immune system and increases your risk of injury.

Intensity (how hard)

F: Low-intensity exercise will not promote weight loss like high-intensity exercise.
Truth: The rate at which calories are burned does not make a difference. The benefit of working out at a lower intensity is that you won't get as tired as quickly.

F: Prayer is only for highly spiritual people.
Truth: Prayer is not just for highly spiritual people. God delights to have you come to Him with your requests. You don't have to be "good enough" to pray.

F: Muscle soreness is a sign of a good workout, "No pain, no gain."
Truth: Exercise is not supposed to hurt. While a little soreness is normal after you start exercising, pain is not. The best relief for muscle soreness is rest, and the best prevention is to be careful not to overdo it in the first place.

F: I must be busy with talking, reading or studying during prayer time.
Truth: Prayer does not mean talking to others, reading or studying. It is not "doing" something. You need to let everything inside you get still. Prayer is a time to have a private audience with the Lord.

F: I should continue working out even if I hurt myself.
Truth: You can still work out after any injury if you modify your workout to exercise around the injury. For example, if you hurt your ankle, it wouldn't be a good idea to jog on it, but you may still be able to do other light exercises in a pool.

Time (how long)

F: I need to spend hours in the gym to see results from an exercise program.
Truth: Even if you don't have time for a formal workout during your day any is better than none. Try to take three 10-minute walks. For strength training, three 20-minute sessions a week will do the job.

F: I must pray for at least one hour at a time.
Truth: You can pray a short, "Lord, help!" or you may shoot a quick prayer of thanks as it comes to you. You can pray as you breathe or you can kneel on your knees and pray for a full 20 minutes. It doesn't need to be a specific time limit.

F: I have to work out for at least 30 minutes at a time for health benefits.
Truth: Any exercise is better than no exercise. Three 10-minute cardiovascular exercise sessions are just as effective for health as one 30-minute bout.

Type (how to exercise)

F: If women lift weights they will bulk up.
Truth: Women have less of the hormone needed to build muscle bulk easily. Very large muscles are most likely not in their genetic potential. Women can't develop huge muscles without spending hours a day lifting very heavy weights.

F: There is only one way to say my prayers.
Truth: There is no "right" way to say prayers, however you may follow the P.A.T.H. to prayer – Praise, Admit, Thank, Help.

F: I need specialized equipment to weight train.
Truth: Ordinary floor exercises that work with the body's own weight can give an excellent and complete muscle workout.

F: I must say the same prayer each day.
Truth: Prayers change as your needs change, your moods change, your heart changes. God does not want a "canned" prayer, but one that is sincere and comes from the heart.

F: I should not start strength training until I am within 25 pounds of my ideal weight.
Truth: Strength training is a cornerstone of weight management. By lifting weights, you build muscle. This extra muscle boosts metabolism, making you burn more calories even when at rest and thereby helping you to lose fat and keep it off.

Chapter 8: Action Plan

Frequency - How often?
Intensity - How hard?
Time - How long?
Type – How to exercise?

Examples:

• I plan to pray every day for 15 minutes in the morning as I walk around the block.
• I plan to participate in a low-impact 60-minute exercise class two times a week.
• I plan to strength train using free weights in my home every other day.

Some ideas to combine active living with a healthy prayer life:

- Pray while walking
- Exercise while watching a Christian program on TV
- Read a Christian magazine/newspaper while working out on a treadmill
- Read the Bible while doing floor warm-up stretches
- Reflect on Scripture during exercise class
- Read a daily prayer from a devotional book before eating
- Listen to the Bible on tape while riding a stationary bike
- Keep a prayer journal of answered prayers

Your turn:

• I plan to

• I plan to

• I plan to

Remember – You need a doctor's approval before beginning an exercise program. Only participate if you are able. Stop if you feel nausea, dizziness, breathlessness or tightness in the chest.

In Closing

I created this book to teach you to move your body to be active every day. I designed it to help you carve a time in your day for prayer.

God's Word, the Bible, tells you that He created you. He loves you and He wants you to love yourself. You are beautiful. He has made everything beautiful (Ecclesiastes 3:11). I developed this program to help you feel good about yourself, no matter what your size. God wants you to be the most beautiful and useful person you can be. Your value is not found in physical appearance but in being a child of God.

Don't just endure life, enjoy it! You can enjoy healthy living – physically and spiritually. Taking care of your body and tending to your spirit adds joy to your life. One cannot be separated from the other. The body, mind and spirit are connected and reflected in your overall health.

There is much that demands your time. Time is a great sacrifice. Where do you want to spend your time? Whichever healthy activities you choose to continue with, make it a daily commitment. May God bless your journey towards improved spiritual and physical health.

For everything God created is good. (1Timothy 4:4a)

About the author

Kimberley Payne is a motivational speaker and writer. Her writing relates raising a family, pursuing a healthy lifestyle, and everyday experiences to building a relationship with God. Kimberley offers practical, guilt-free tips on improving spiritual and physical health. Visit her website www.kimberleypayne.com

*

Did you enjoy this book? Please take a moment to write a review. Share the blessings.

Books in the Fit for Faith Series

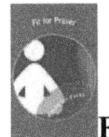

Fit for Prayer
Learn how to fit prayer and physical activity into your daily routine. The book unites physical health and spiritual health to help you lose weight and develop a deeper relationship with God.
Buy your copy! http://bit.ly/FitForPrayer

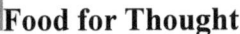

Food for Thought
Find out how to nourish your body and spirit through healthy eating and Bible study. Just as eating healthy foods nourishes your body, Bible study nourishes your spirit. You will learn practical suggestions and scriptural guidance to achieve your goals.
Buy your copy! http://bit.ly/Food-For-Thought

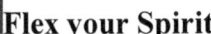

Flex your Spirit
Discover a new way to express yourself with God through journal writing and stretching. Learn how to recharge your physical and emotional health through stretching activities for your body and spirit.
Buy your copy! http://bit.ly/FlexYourSpirit

Collect them all!

Fit for Faith – 7 weeks to improved spiritual and physical health combines all three books into **one workbook** plus adds health & fitness myths, a home fitness test, strength training and stretching exercises, and a food diary. The workbook also includes a 49-day plan to empower you to improve your spiritual and physical health!

Buy your copy today! http://bit.ly/FitForFaithBook

Women of Strength – a devotional to improve spiritual and physical health includes a devotional article, question & answer, reflection, prayer, Bible truth, top tips, praise moves and a challenge to apply active living.

Buy your copy today! http://bit.ly/WomenOfStrength

Online Courses

www.kimberleypayne.com/e-courses/

Do you want to make the disciplines of exercise, prayer, healthy eating, Bible study, stretching and journal writing a part of your daily routine? All three books are also available as **virtual home-study courses**.

Home study
Watch the 7 video tutorials on your own time. Watch them all in a row, one a day or one a week. It's entirely up to you!

Spiritual component
Learn about prayer, Bible study, and journal writing to connect on a deeper level with God.

Physical component
Learn about healthy eating, cardio and strength training, and stretching exercises to incorporate into your day.

Support group
Ask questions, express concerns, and receive encouragement from other women.

Not sure if you want to commit to a full 7-module course?
Then take just module one for free!
Visit www.kimberleypayne.com/free-programs to register!

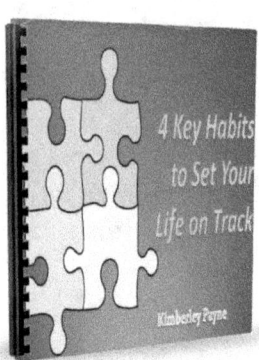

<u>Free Report</u> Reveals…
The 4 Key Habits to Set your Life on Track

7 health & fitness experts share their top spiritual & physical health tips.

Learn quick tips to improve your daily habits in Bible study, eating healthy, exercise and prayer.

Visit <u>www.kimberleypayne.com/free-report</u>
to download your free report today!